AESTHETICS: IT'S BULKING SEASON!

FOLLOW US ON TWITTER: @AestheticsBooks

INTRODUCTION

To be quite frank with you guys, I never expected my first work, "Aesthetics 101", to be the success that it was. If it wasn't for my great supporters I would not have published this second book. Respect!

Now let's get back on topic. If you read the first installment in the 'Aesthetics' series, you would be aware of my style and aware of the fact that I tend to avoid going deep into scientific detail especially since this is a bodybuilding guide and not a textbook. I will have to cover some basics though so that you would have a general idea at least.

There are many bodybuilding myths that say how it is possible for one to lose fat and gain muscle simultaneously. While our bodies aren't able to do both "simultaneously", alternating between periods of cutting and periods of bulking throughout a given week (known as carbohydrate cycling, which was covered in Aesthetics 101) makes it a possibility. However, some people find it more efficient to go through separate periods of bulking and cutting to reach their goals in a quicker and timelier fashion. In this guide, the focus will be on bulking.

When a bodybuilder goes through a bulking phase, he typically goes through with it during the winter season since shirtless times at the beach are minimal to nonexistent. The reason for this is that fat gain is inevitable during a bulk. However, this guide will teach you ways to keep that fat gain minimal.

During a bulk, one must modify his diet so that calories consumed are higher than calories burnt by the body. By eating more than your overall caloric expenditure, these extra calories will be stored by the body as either fat or muscle. What determines this outcome if the cleanliness and quality of food the bodybuilder eats. People who go on a "dirty bulk" and eat anything and everything in sight end up gaining a little of muscle and much fat, which gives them the bloated look.

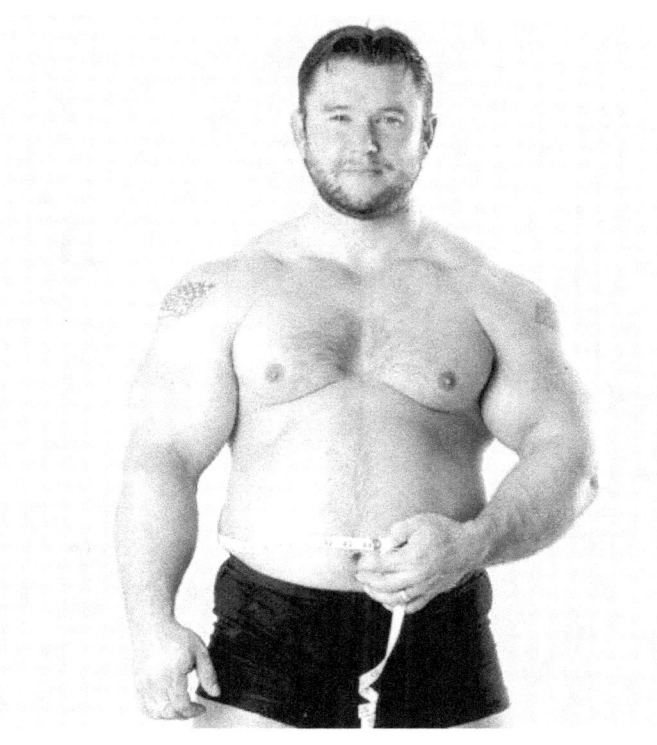

Unless you want to look like that, never attempt to dirty bulk!

This guide will focus on adding 3500 calories above maintenance per week (500 calories per day), which will add about 1-1.5 pounds of lean muscle per week. If you like what you hear and are willing to give up those dreams of making multiple trips to McDonald's to get by, read on!

WHO IS BULKING FOR?

You must remember that in order for you to bulk and maintain muscular definition, you must be lean to begin with. I am not an advocate of bulking without regard to definition and then cutting down afterwards. I prefer to look lean and ripped year round rather than acquiring aesthetics on a seasonal basis.

My personal recommendation is to avoid bulking if you have any body fat percentage above 10%. Other experts set the threshold to 12%, but I would much rather maintain a solid six pack throughout the duration of my bulk. This is a personal preference, however. If you are fine with sacrificing definition for a period of time then by all means, feel free to bulk at whatever body fat percentage you desire!

The most ideal way for you to measure your body fat percentage would be for you to visit your local health center (or gym if they offer such services) and take a body composition evaluation in which they use calipers to accurately measure your body fat percentage. If you do not have access to such services, here's a good way to get a close estimate:

1. Measure your weight in pounds. If you only know your weight in kilograms, multiply that number by 2.205. I will use my own measurements as an example to this formula. I weigh 75 kilograms (75 x 2.205 = 165 pounds)

2. Multiply your weight in pounds by 1.082 (165 x 1.082 = 178.53)

3. Add 94.42 to the resulting number (178.53 + 94.42 = 272.95)

4. Measure your waist girth using a measuring tape. Make sure that the measurement is taken at the belly button (navel) level. My measurement is 29 cm.

5. Multiply your waist girth by 4.15 (29 x 4.15 = 120.35)

6. Subtract the result found in step 5 from the result found in step 3 (272.95 – 120.35 = 152.6) This number represents your lean body mass (LBM), which is the weight of your body components without taking fat into account.

7. Subtract your LBM from your total body mass (TBM), which you found in step 1 (165 – 152.6 = 12.4)

8. Multiply the result by 100 (12.4 x 100 = 1240)

9. Divide the result by your TBM (1240 / 165 = 7.5% body fat)

DIET

As I stated earlier, in order to bulk and put on lean muscle mass you must add an average of 500 calories above maintenance.

To calculate your daily caloric intake, use the following formula:

1. First, we must calculate BMR (basic metabolic rate). This is the formula for men (I hope no woman is attempting to bulk using this book!)

   BMR = 66.47 + (13.75 x (weight (lb) / 2.2)) + (5 x ((height (in) x 2.54))

   – (6.75 x age (years))

   = 66.47 + (13.75 x (165 / 2.2)) + (5 x ((70 x 2.54)) – (6.75 x 19) =1858 calories

2. Multiply your BMR by your activity level (we will use the "active" classification since we are actively lifting as bodybuilders; the activity level for this is 1.7)

   = 1858 calories x 1.7 = 3159 calories

3. Add 500 calories above maintenance! (3159 + 500 = 3659 calories)

Now that you have your daily caloric needs, all you will need to do to create the perfect meal plan if distribute your calories in the following ratio: 50/40/10, with 50% allotted to carbohydrates, 40% to protein, and 10% to fats. You must choose from a range of healthy foods (complex carbohydrates, lean meats, and unsaturated fats). Here are some meal plan examples to get you started:

The following sample meal plans are designed for an individual weighing 180 lb. Be sure to adjust this diet to your own weight before using it!

Sample Day 1 (Workout Day)

Breakfast:

- 1 scoop whey protein, 1 scoop casein protein
- 1 apple
- 3 eggs (with yolks)
- 3 egg whites
- 2 cups oatmeal (measure before cooking; cook in water)

  Note: I add the protein (chocolate is my favorite) to the oatmeal since it tastes horrible in water alone!

Mid-Morning Snack:

- 1 cup Raisin Bran cereal with 1 cup skim milk
- 1 scoop whey protein

Lunch:

- 4 slices whole wheat bread
- 6 oz roast beef
- 1 slice low fat American cheese
- 2 cups spinach

Pre-Workout (30-45 minutes prior):

- 1 scoop whey protein
- 1 cup oatmeal (in water)

Post-Workout (immediately after workout):

- 2 scoops whey protein
- 2.5 cups Gatorade

Dinner:

- 6 oz turkey breast
- 1 cup (cooked) brown rice
- 1 cup broccoli

Pre-Bed:

- 1 cup low fat cottage cheese
- 1 tablespoon natural peanut butter

TOTALS: 3,879 calories, 356g protein, 399g carbs, 80g fat

Sample Day 2 (Workout Day)

Breakfast:

- 1 scoop whey protein, 1 scoop casein protein
- 1 cup oatmeal (in water)
- 3 eggs (with yolks)
- 3 egg whites
- 3 slices lean turkey bacon
- 2 whole wheat English muffins

Mid-Morning Snack:

- 1 cup Raisin Bran cereal with 1 cup skim milk
- 1 scoop whey protein

Lunch:

- 2 whole wheat tortillas
- 8 oz deli turkey
- ½ cup spinach
- 6 oz hummus

Pre-Workout (30-45 minutes prior):

- 1 scoop whey protein
- 1 orange

Post-Workout (immediately after workout):

- 1 scoop whey protein, 1 scoop casein protein
- 1 medium-sized plain white bagel
- 1 tablespoon strawberry jam

Dinner:

- 9 oz salmon
- 1 cup brown rice
- 1 cup broccoli
- 2 cups spinach

Pre-Bed:

- 1 scoop casein protein
- 1 oz almonds

TOTALS: 4,060 calories, 355g protein, 396g carbs, 108g fat

As you may know, caloric intake should be slightly lower on rest days due to the lack of pre and post workout meals. You should eat at around your maintenance calories on days when you have no workouts (1-2 days per week at most). Here is a sample meal plan for a rest day. Keep in mind that the calories cut down on rest days come from carbohydrates while protein and fat remain the same.

Sample Day 3 (Rest Day)

Breakfast:

- 1 scoop whey protein, 1 scoop casein protein
- 2 cups watermelon
- 3 eggs (with yolks)
- 3 egg whites
- 3 slices lean turkey bacon
- 2 whole wheat English muffins

Mid-Morning Snack:

- 1 scoop casein protein
- ½ cup granola

Lunch:

- 2 beef patties (90% lean)
- 1 slice low fat American cheese
- 1 whole wheat hamburger bun
- ½ cup spinach

Afternoon Snack:

- 6 celery stalks
- 1 tablespoon natural peanut butter

Dinner:

- 9 oz tilapia
- 1 cup brown rice
- 2 tablespoons salsa
- 2 cups spinach

Pre-Bed:

- 1 scoop casein protein
- 1 oz walnuts

TOTALS: 3,300 calories, 311g protein, 253g carbs, 115g fat

TRAINING

The training aspect of achieving aesthetics is much more important in bulking than it is in cutting (and the diet is less important!), therefore you should ensure that you never miss a workout since each one is fundamental to your muscle growth and those last 1 or 2 reps may make the difference in the growth of some quality lean muscle mass!

I recommend and found a 4-day split to be the most effective while bulking. Light cardio (walking at a brisk pace for 20-30 minutes) should be done on rest days or after your workout to keep your heart in a healthy state and to keep that fat off!

It is also recommended that you split your workout evenly throughout the week rather than do them all on consecutive days. Here is an example layout of my bulking workout regimen:

The glossary of all exercises is in the back of this book. Also, the reason for the lower reps with each set is because you are expected to increase the performed weight with each set.

Monday (Shoulders and Triceps):

Shoulders:

- Smith machine shoulder press (4 sets x 12,10,8,6 reps)

- Dumbbell lateral raise (4 sets x 12,10,8,6 reps)

- Dumbbell Reverse Fly (4 sets x 12,10,8,6 reps)

- Dumbbell Shrugs (4 sets x 12,10,8,6 reps)

Triceps:

- Lying tricep extension (3 sets x 10,8,6 reps)

- One arm cable extension (3 sets x 10,8,6 reps)

- One arm dumbbell extension (3 sets x 10,8,6 reps)

Tuesday (Back and Abs):

Back:

- Wide grip pull-up (4 sets x 12,10,8,6 reps)

- Close grip pulldown (4 sets x 12,10,8,6 reps)

- One arm dumbbell row (4 sets x 12,10,8,6 reps)

- Bent over dumbbell row (4 sets x 12,10,8,6 reps)

Abs:

- Reverse crunch (3 sets x 20 reps)

- Crunch (3 sets x 20 reps)

Wednesday (Cardio; 30 minute walk at brisk pace)

Thursday (Chest and Biceps):

Chest:

- Incline dumbbell press (4 sets x 12,10,8,6 reps)

- Bench press (4 sets x 12,10,8,6 reps)

- Incline dumbbell fly (4 sets x 12,10,8,6 reps)

- Cable crossover (4 sets x 12,10,8,6 reps)

Biceps:

- Incline dumbbell curl (3 sets x 10,8,6 reps)

- Preacher curl (3 sets x 10,8,6 reps)

- Standing hammer curl (3 sets x 10,8,6 reps)

Friday (Legs and Abs):

Legs:

- Squats (4 sets x 12,10,8,6 reps)

- Leg press (4 sets x 12,10,8,6 reps)

- Leg extension (4 sets x 12,10,8,6 reps)

- Stiff leg deadlift (4 sets x 12,10,8,6 reps)

- Seated calf raise (4 sets x 12,10,8,6 reps)

- Standing calf raise (4 sets x 12,10,8,6 reps)

Abs:

- Reverse crunch (3 sets x 20 reps)

- Crunch (3 sets x 20 reps)

Saturday (Cardio; 30 minute walk at brisk pace)

Sunday (REST)

SUPPLEMENTATION

It is not necessary to supplement vitamins and other crucial nutrients (zinc, magnesium, etc.) while on a bulk since your diet is already rich in all of these nutrients. A general multivitamin could be used if desired, however.

Here is a list of the supplements I support the use of during the bulking phase:

Pre-Workout:

- N.O. Xplode 2.0

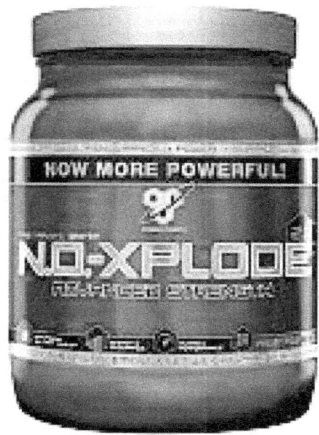

Whey Protein:

- Gold Standard100% Whey by Optimum Nutrition

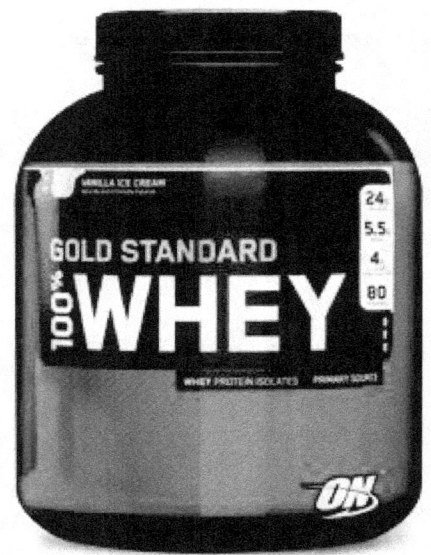

- Syntha-6 by BSN

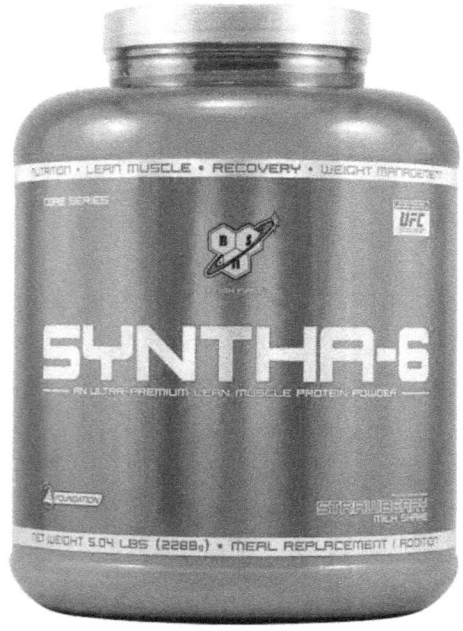

Multivitamins:

- One a Day

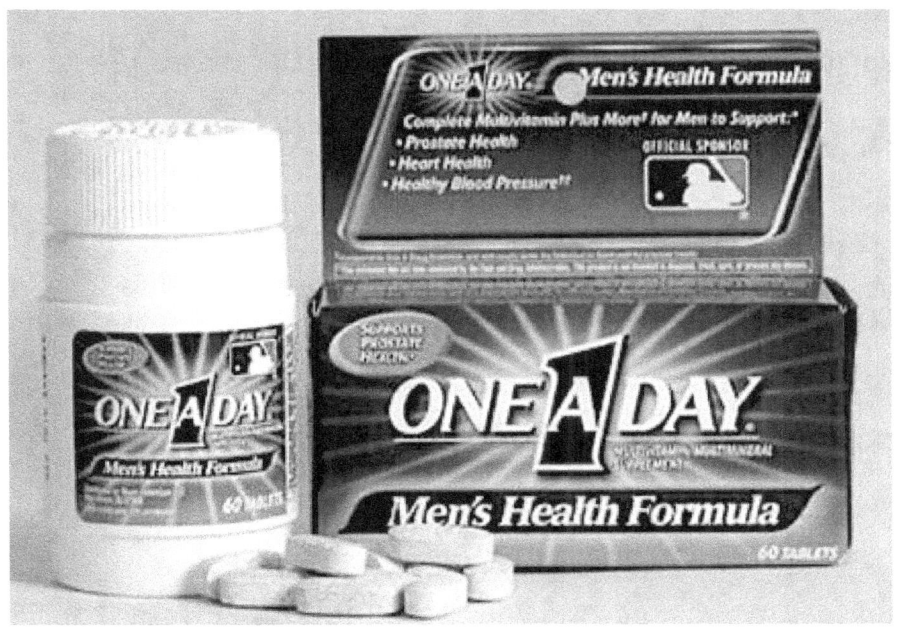

- Opti-Men

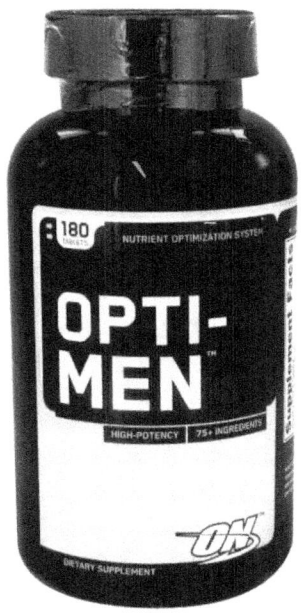

REST

Sleep is very crucial in the muscle-building process. One should aim to get no less than 6 hours of sleep a night and no more than 8 hours. I feel that my performance peaks when I get my hours of sleep within that range and getting any less or any more sleep leaves me feeling cranky and moody.

You should also focus on getting your first meal of the day immediately after waking up to replenish your stores and focus on getting your last meal in less than an hour before bedtime to avoid getting your body into a fasted state during sleep, which may lead to muscle loss.

CONCLUSION

That's all there is to bulking, folks! It's relatively simple and straight-forward, but you must have the motivation and dedication to get all of those CLEAN calories in and stay away from that devilish "dirty bulk" which will give you nothing but a nasty gut!

I will be glad to assist you guys with any questions you may have and would love to hear about your progress in the bulking phase. Feel free to post on our Twitter page @AestheticsBooks or email me personally at njk36@drexel.edu

ENJOY THE RIDE!

GET RIPPED OR DIE MIRIN!

GLOSSARY OF EXERCISES

Smith Machine Shoulder Press

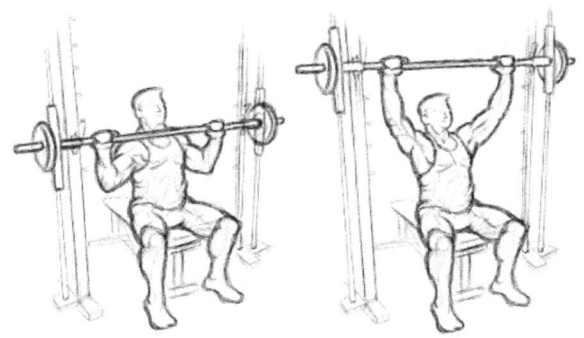

Dumbbell Lateral Raise

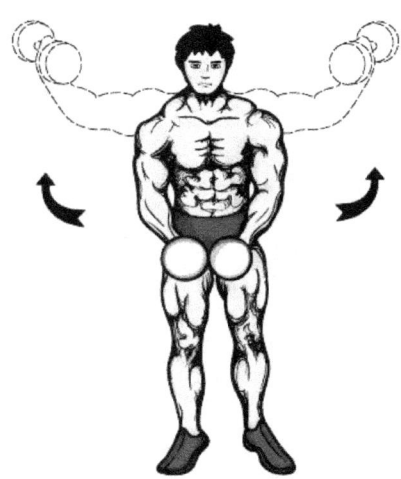

Dumbbell Reverse Fly

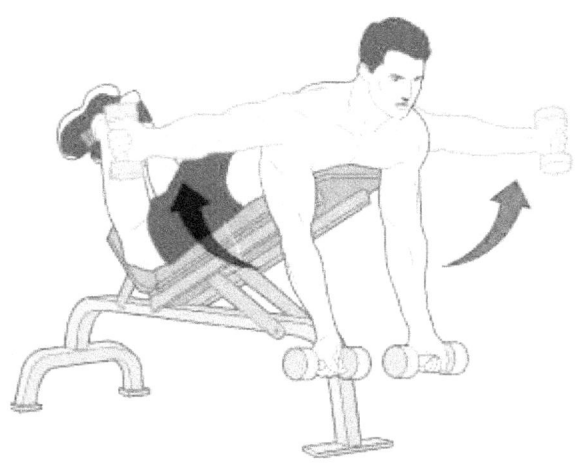

Dumbbell Shrugs

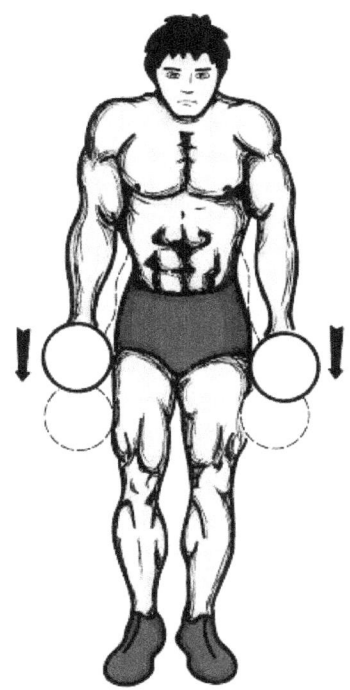

Lying Tricep Extension

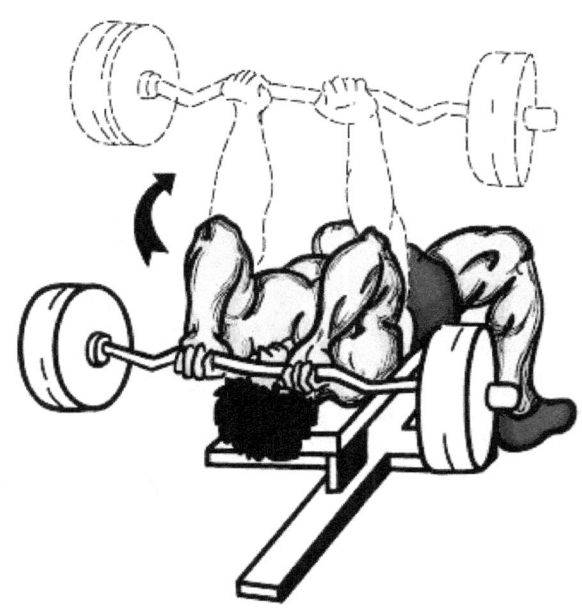

One Arm Cable Extension

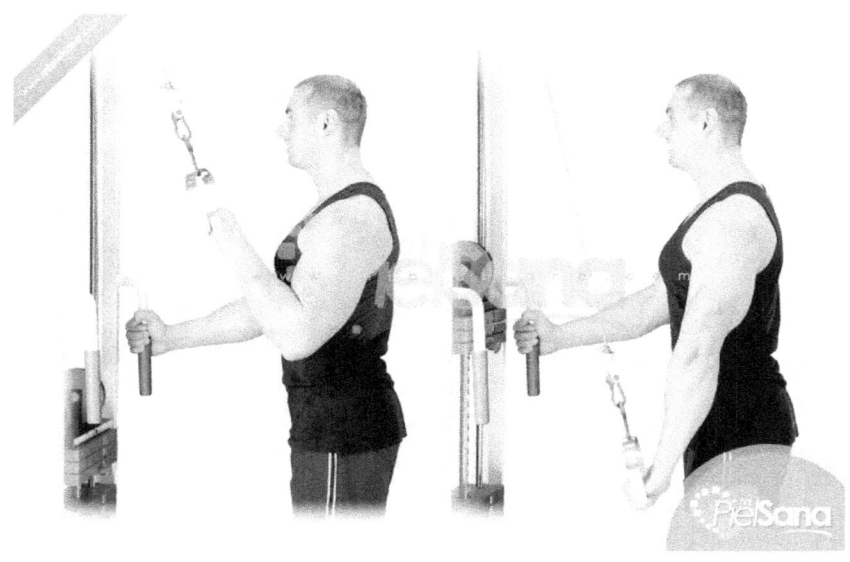

One Arm Dumbbell Extension

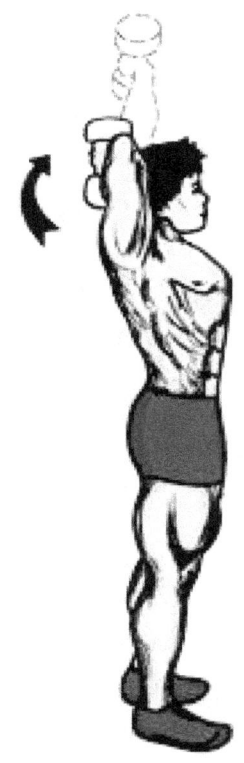

Building-Muscle101.com

Wide Grip Pullup

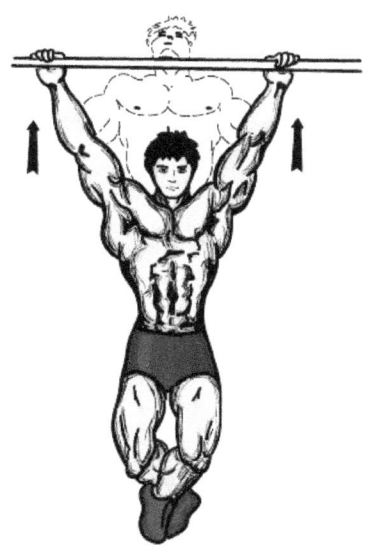

Close Grip Pulldown

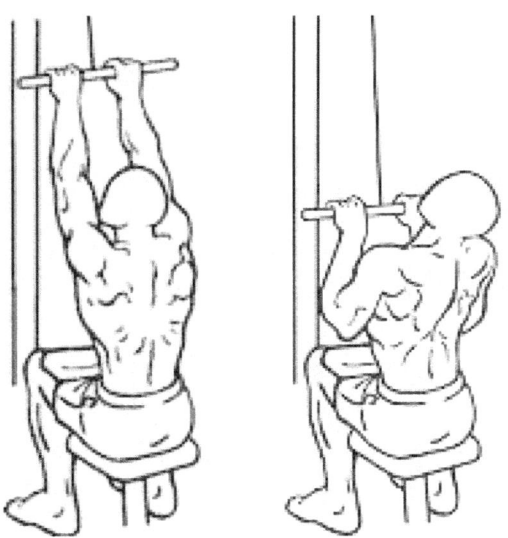

One Arm Dumbbell Row

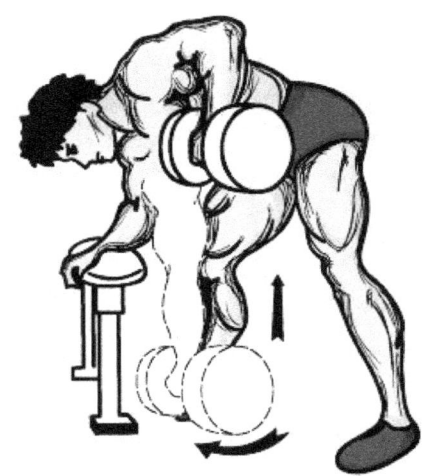

Incline Dumbbell Press

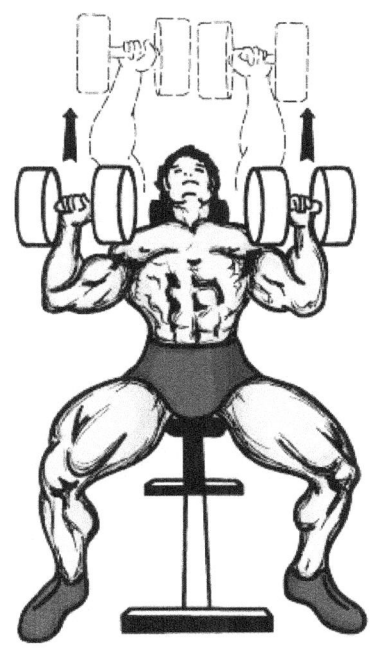

Bench Press

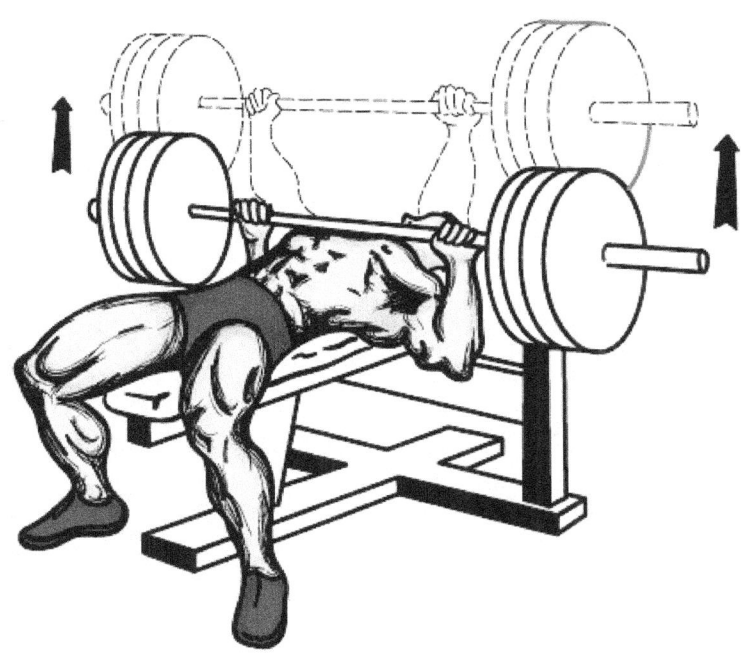

Incline Dumbbell Fly

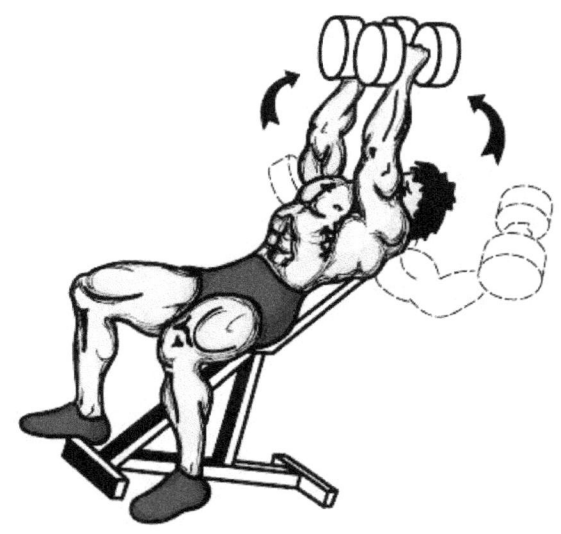

Cable Crossover

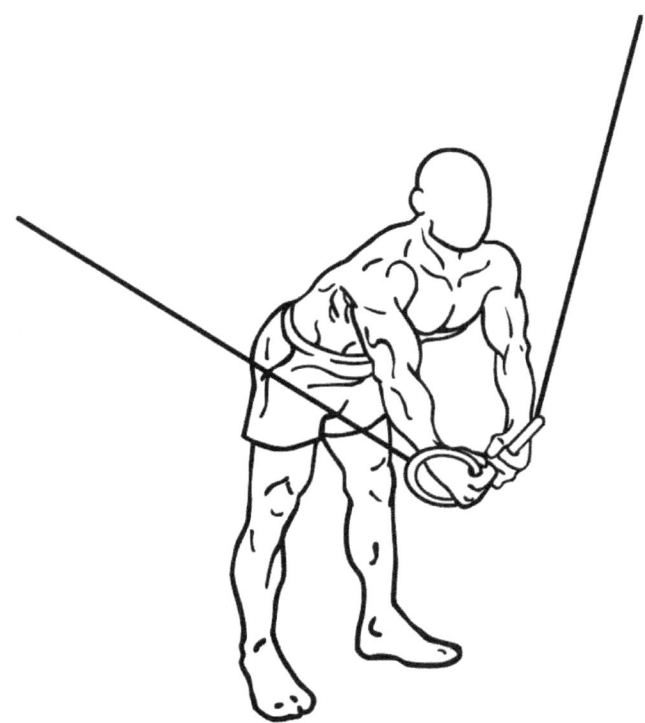

Incline Dumbbell Curl

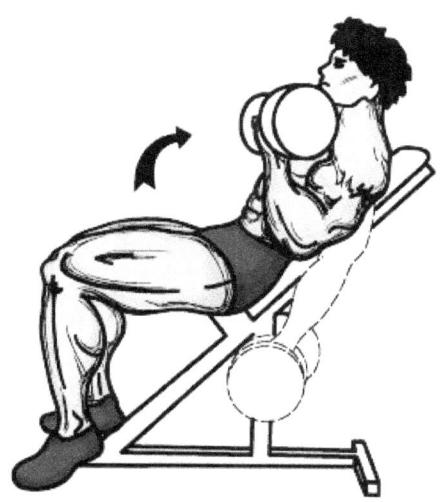

Preacher Curl

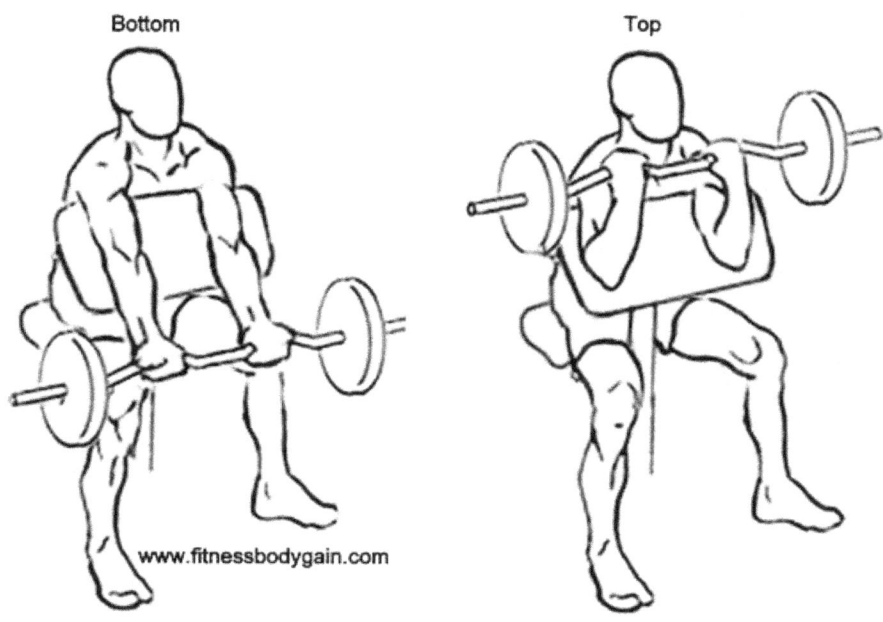

Bottom

Top

www.fitnessbodygain.com

Standing Hammer Curl

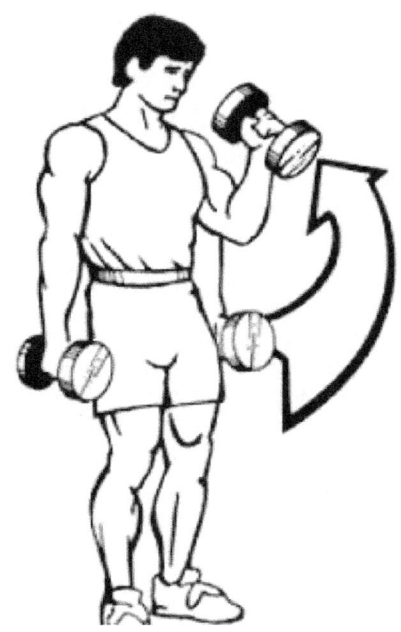

Squat

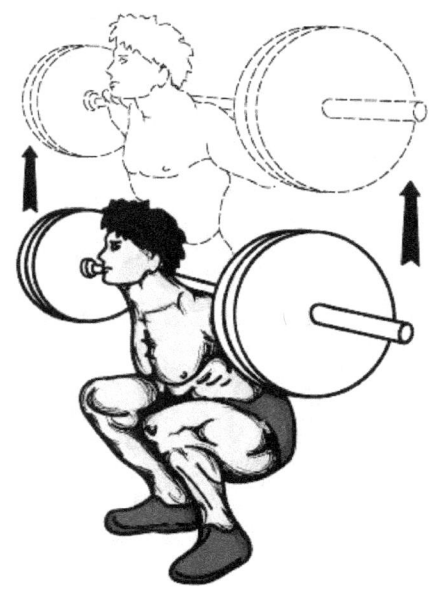

Leg Press

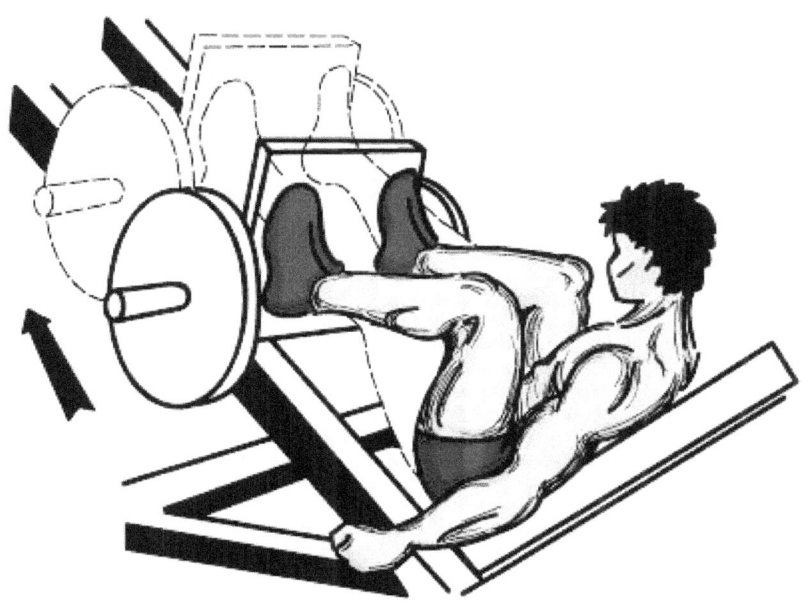

Leg Extension

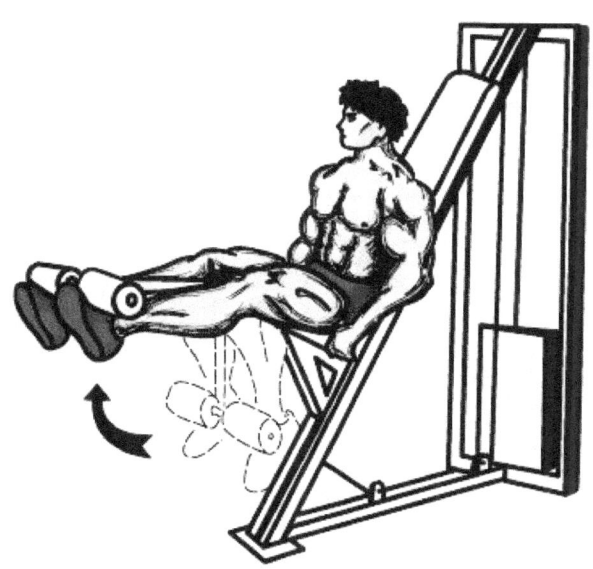

Stiff Leg Deadlift

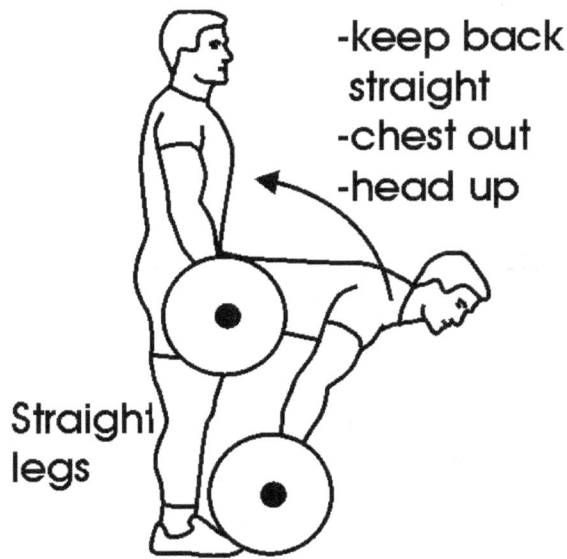

-keep back
 straight
-chest out
-head up

Straight
legs

Seated Calf Raise

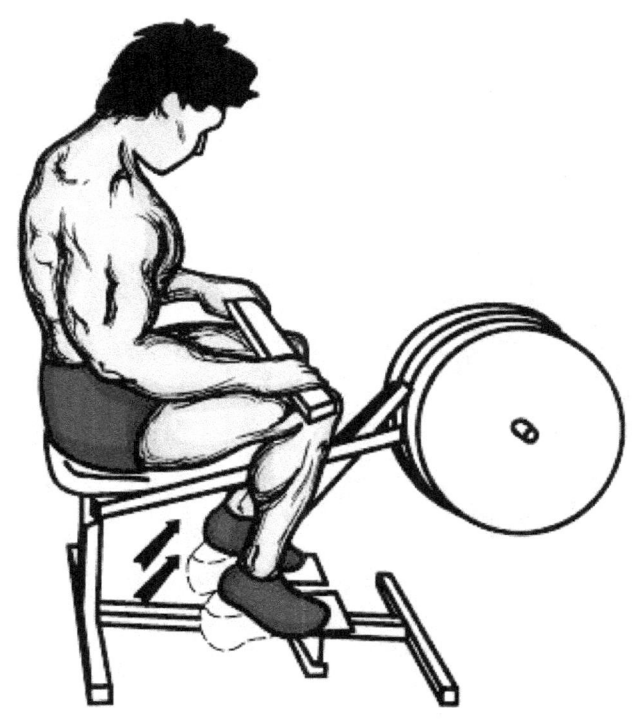

Standing Calf Raise

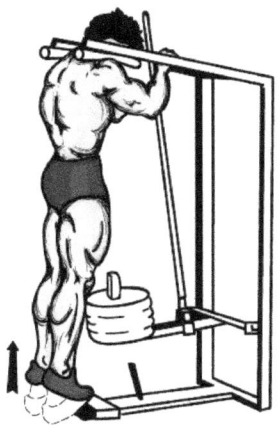

Crunch

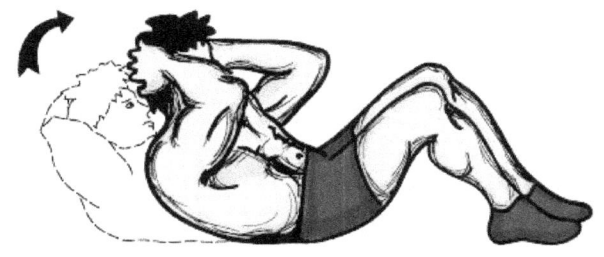

Reverse Crunch

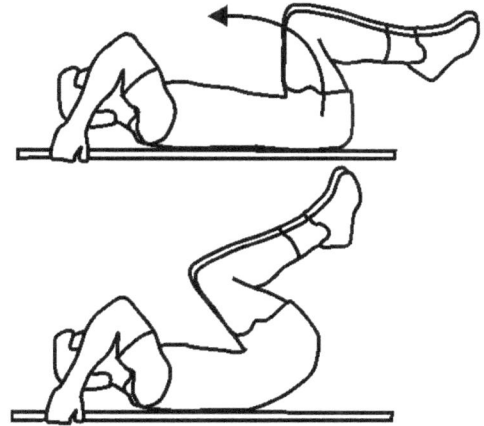